THE COMPLETE GUIDE TO HAIR REMOVAL FOR WOMEN

BY LORI WEINTRAUB

Disclaimer

The information in this book is based on my personal observations and assessments over the course of my 30+ year career. These are strictly my opinions with regard to what I have seen in my treatment room. I am sharing my knowledge and experience as it relates to my work. Readers are fully responsible for all decisions made with regard to the hair removal methods they choose to use as well as their choice of a hair removal practitioner when applicable.

About Lori

Lori Weintraub has been working in the field of permanent hair removal known as Electrolysis (the "un-laser") for over 30 years.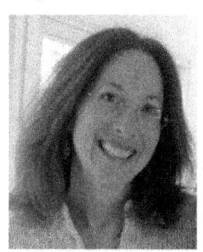

In addition to being a Master Electrologist, she is also a Licensed Esthetician with a comprehensive knowledge of the skin.

She is honored to have helped hundreds of women improve their appearances as well as their self-esteem.

Visit her websites at:

www.hairremovalbylori.com

www.integrativeskincaring.com

Email: info@hairremovalbylori.com

Dedication

I dedicate this book to all the wonderful women who have entrusted me with their skin and unwanted hairs over the past 30+ years.

Within the confines of my treatment room, they have shared their stories with me. Many have expressed that I have changed their lives by liberating them of their embarrassment.

I wonder how many realize that they have made a difference in my life as well.

Contents

Introduction

In my 30+ years in the field of hair removal, I have witnessed firsthand the frustration, confusion and desperation of women who are plagued with excessive amounts of embarrassing hair growth on their faces as well as their bodies.

At my initial consultation with a prospective client, I ask a lot of questions about their hair growth issue:

- What specific area of the face or body requires treatment?
- How long have you had this problem?
- What measures have you taken to deal with it?
- Is your menstrual cycle normal?
- Are you under a doctor's care?
- What, if any, prescription medications are you taking?

- Do you have hair on the upper chest or on your breasts?
- Have you ever been tested for a hormonal imbalance?

It is not uncommon for women to wipe away tears as tell their story.

Some style their hair in such a way as to hide the whiskers that are on their cheeks and sides of the face.

Others use the "thinking stance" while conversing so that their hand is cupped over the chin and part of the lip.

Many stand in front of their bathroom mirror applying thick layers of foundation to cover up any visible hair growth.

So many women pluck and tweeze extensively to the point that the skin becomes inflamed and damaged.

Bright light, sunshine and close personal contact are known to cause anxiety as the hairs are more readily seen.

Teenage girls are often teased at school or hear whispered conversations as other students point and stare.

These are just a mere few of the many stories that I have heard through the years.

My goal in writing this book is to provide you with the facts as I know them. Use this guide to help you to sort through the various hair removal options that are available.

♥ *Lori*

The History of Hair Removal

Throughout history, women have resorted to using drastic measures to rid themselves of excess body hair.

Drawings discovered on cave walls reveal that the cavemen (and probably cavewomen when they viewed their reflection in a pool of water!) scraped hair off their faces with sharpened pieces of flint. Seashells pressed together to form tweezer-like tools were also known to be used.

Depilatory hair removal creams were concocted as far back as 4000 B.C. These creams contained a combination of harsh chemicals such as arsenic.

In ancient Egypt, the Pharaoh's wives removed hair from their bodies with a sticky goop made of honey, oil and lemon.

Threading has been around for hundreds of years. It is believed that women removed their body hair before their wedding day as this was considered to be a rite of passage.

In the middle ages, a high hairline was a sign of aristocracy. For that reason, women would pluck their hairline back about an inch or more to stay fashionable.

As fashion evolved during the 1900s, women were showing more visible skin. This required them to shave their legs as well as their underarms.

Early Hollywood movies were also influential in style setting. Eyebrow pencil was used to create thin, exaggerated brows after all existing hairs were tweezed out.

The razor manufacturer Gillette™ created an advertising campaign directed at women. This was a boom for their sales as women raced to the nearest store to purchase razors so that their skin would be smooth, silky and hair free.

Hormonal Hair Growth

Many women visit my office after their physician has diagnosed them with a hormonal imbalance. Polycystic Ovary Syndrome, also referred to as PCOS, is one of the most common of these imbalances.

Others, who are disheartened by increasing amounts of newly appearing hairs, may be unaware of the cause.

As a hair removal expert, I am experienced at observing hair growth patterns which may indicate an underlying medical condition that is stimulating hairs to grow in excess.

In addition to facial hair, there are other clues that suggest hormonal issues, such as:

- Acne breakouts on the cheeks
- Thinning appearance of the "good hair" on the head at the temples

- Visible hair on the upper chest and cleavage
- Long and abundant growth on the arms

Questions that I may ask:

- Do you have hair growth on your breasts or around your nipples?
- Is your menstrual cycle normal?
- Have you seen any hairs on your upper back or shoulders?

After my assessment, I may suggest that the client discuss these issues with her gynecologist. Her doctor will probably want to order blood work to determine if there is an underlying hormonal imbalance.

Hirsutism

Hirsutism is the term used to describe a woman who has an excessive amount of hair on the face and body. It does not mean that the woman has a disease or illness.

Genetics often plays a large role in the amount and location of unwanted hairs. Throughout the years, I have treated many mothers, daughters and sisters. When working on them, I often see the same exact pattern of growth between these family members.

Ethnicity is also a contributing factor in how much hair a woman has. For example, women of Mediterranean descent tend to have more hair than those of Asian descent.

When a woman suddenly notices an increase in the amount of hair along with thickening and darkening, it would be prudent to bring this to the attention of a physician.

Androgens

Some women with PCOS (polycystic ovary syndrome) have elevated levels of androgens. Androgens are hormones that are produced in the adrenal glands and the ovaries.

When androgens levels are high there might be an increase of unsightly hair growth on a woman's face and body. The tiny "peach fuzz" hairs may be altered by the androgen influence. As a result, these formally invisible hairs may begin to grow darker, thicker and longer.

A woman with androgen-sensitive hair growth patterns will see excess hairs, as follows:

Most Common

- Upper lip
- Chin and neck
- Breasts

- Lower back
- Lower abdomen

Less Common

- Upper chest region
- Upper abdomen
- Upper back

Androgen-sensitive hair growth is one of the many symptoms that women with PCOS deal with. In order to minimize future increases in new hair growth, it is important to consult with a physician in this regard. After testing, your doctor may determine that you require some type of hormonal therapy.

It is unlikely; however, that visible hairs already present will be reduced or minimized.

How to Use this Guide

Each heading will highlight a particular hair removal product type or method.

This book has been designed so that you, the user, will have an easy way to reference information.

Since many products and/or methods function in similar ways, you may find that the same exact wording has been repeated in multiple categories.

You can read all the pages, or simply go directly to the heading that you are most interested in. Perhaps this will be a product or service that is currently in use, or something you are considering as your next step.

Hair Vocabulary

Vellus – These are the very fine hairs that are generally invisible and give the skin a soft coating. They are often times referred to as "peach fuzz." Women have this type of hair on the face, chest, stomach and back.

Terminal – This type of hair is generally darker in color and thicker in texture than the above-mentioned vellus hairs.

Terminal hair growth is found on the legs, underarms and in the bikini area. A woman's "crowning glory" consists entirely of terminal hair growth.

Women with hormonal imbalances (such as Polycystic Ovary Syndrome) will notice more terminal-like hair growth on their faces. There may also be visible hair on the breasts, upper chest, stomach, shoulders and back. Arms may grow longer, denser hairs as well.

Note: Please keep these terms in mind while you read through this guide.

The difference between the two types of hairs -- **vellus** and **terminal** -- is important to your understanding of how various hair removal methods work.

Temporary Measures

This is a huge category. I will address the product types and methods that I am currently aware of.

Keep in mind that all temporary measures have the disadvantage of requiring continual maintenance since the hair always grows back. In some cases, <u>a number of these methods also increase hair growth.</u>

Many manufacturers use clever marketing phrases which persuade women into believing that their product can reduce or eliminate unwanted hairs forever.

Please note that there may be products available outside the United States that I am not familiar with. Additionally, newer product types may appear in the marketplace after the publication of this guide.

Bleaching Creams

Bleaching creams are typically packaged as a two-part product. The first part is a jar of cream and the second part is the powdered bleach.

The user is directed to mix equal amounts of the cream and the powder in order to create a paste. The paste is then applied to the area requiring bleaching. Seven to ten minutes is standard for the bleaching process to be completed.

Important: Be sure to read and follow the manufacturer's directions, since they may be different from what I have mentioned above.

Pros: Bleaching lightens unsightly hairs and helps to minimize their appearance. This is a simple process which does not affect the hair growth in any way. It makes it appear less visible because the hairs will turn whitish-blonde.

Cons: The bleach may cause a reaction in individuals with extremely sensitive skin.

Always test the mixture on the inside of the forearm and wait 24 hours to determine if there is a reaction. If there is no redness or irritation present, it would be safe to use it on the face.

To first time users, I recommend mixing a bit less of the powdered bleach than directed on the package and applying it for only half the amount of time. This would be a good test to see how the skin on the face reacts. The second time around you can leave it on longer and mix it full strength, if you feel that your skin will handle it without issue.

When the cream sits on the skin, it may sting and itch. You will need to be tolerant of this sensation in order to use the product properly.

Additionally, you might smell the scent of the bleach when it is applied to the lip area. If so, try to breathe out of your mouth instead of your nose to minimize the odor.

Depilatory Hair Removal Creams

Depilatories are generally designed for use on areas of the body such as arms and legs; although there are also specific ones available for the face. When the depilatory cream is applied to the skin, the chemicals in the product dissolve the hair at the surface.

First time users should test the product on the inner arm and wait 24 hours to determine if there is a reaction.

These products are sold at chain drug stores and supermarkets. They are available in gel, cream, aerosol, roll-on and powder form.

They are scented to cover up the chemical odor in order to make them more user-friendly.

Pros: Depilatories can be used on arms and legs as long as your skin does not have a sensitivity or allergic reaction to the chemicals in the product. Unlike shaving which cuts the hair at the skin's surface, the depilatory sinks slightly into the depression at the pore opening. For this reason, the skin will feel smoother and less stubbly than it would after shaving.

Cons: It is my opinion that you <u>should not use depilatories on your face, neck, chest or stomach.</u> Even if you have terminal hairs in these areas, there is also a covering of fine vellus hairs. When these tiny hairs are tampered with, they will be stimulated to grow back longer, darker and more abundant over time.

Dermaplane

Dermaplaning is a type of esthetic facial procedure that deeply exfoliates the skin as well as removes any surface hair growth.

This service is typically performed by an esthetician (licensed skin care therapist) who holds a scalpel at a 45 degree angle in order to remove the top most superficial layers of the skin. To avoid nicks and cuts, the skin must be held tautly during the procedure.

Pros: It helps to smooth rough skin and is a form of exfoliation that functions similar to a chemical peel, but without the chemicals.

Cons: If this is not done by an experienced technician with a steady hand, there is the risk of nicks and scrapes.

Additionally, the action of the scalpel against the skin will result in the removal of all the vellus hairs on the face. While this may seem desirable, those fine little vellus hairs will be stimulated to grow darker, longer and denser. If you are determined to have a peel, I suggest that you consider an alternative method.

Epilator

An epilator is a handheld device that looks similar in appearance to that of a battery operated shaver. Unlike a shaver that cuts the hair at the skin's surface, the epilator houses a coil-like mechanism which grabs and pulls the hair out of the skin as it rotates. Some models use rotating metal plates to grab and extract the hairs instead of a coil.

Pros: Epilating can be done on any area of the body and easily removes large amounts of hairs as the device glides along the skin's surface. The epilator action pulls the entire hair out of the skin from the root. It will take several days to a few weeks for all the hairs to be visible on the surface again. The reward is smooth skin that stays hair-free longer than shaving.

Cons: Although the action is similar to that of tweezing, it hurts more because so many hairs are being pulled out at the same time. Hairs must be at least 1/8" long in order to be grabbed by the device.

Due to the pulling action of the epilator, some of the thicker hairs may break off at the surface. If this happens, ingrown hairs often develop. I would suggest using a loofah with a gel cleanser or a scrub to gently exfoliate the skin between epilating sessions. This will help to keep the hairs growing freely out of the skin.

It is my opinion that <u>epilating should not be done on the face, neck, chest or stomach.</u> Even if you have terminal hairs in these areas, there is also a covering of fine vellus hairs. When these tiny hairs are tampered with, they will be stimulated to grow back longer, darker and more abundant over time.

Facial Buffer

This item uses a mitt with a sandpaper-like substance at the base. The user is instructed to rub the skin in different directions with the facial buffer as a way of wearing the hair down to the skin surface.

This may work with some of the finer hairs, but the thicker hairs would require numerous passes with vigorous stroking in order to break them down.

Pros: Your skin will be exfoliated with the use of the facial buffer.

Cons: Overuse will create skin irritation and inflammation. In some individuals with darker complexions, pigmentation issues are likely to develop over time.

It is my opinion that facial buffer should not be used on the face at all. Even if you have some dark terminal hairs, there is also a covering of fine vellus hairs. When these tiny hairs are tampered with, they will be stimulated to grow back longer, darker and more abundant over time.

Grooming Razors

These razors are typically marketed for use on the eyebrows. Many women also use them on areas of the face where there is excess hair growth.

Pros: When used slightly above the skin's surface, they are capable of shortening some of the longer hairs without tampering with the fine vellus ones.

Cons: Using the grooming razor to remove all the hairs on the entire face, will eventually cause the finer hairs to grow back thicker and more abundant over time. Continual maintenance will be required to keep the hairs under control.

Heat and Light Devices
No!No!™ | Finishing Touch YES™ | etc.

The above-mentioned devices purport to use heat or light technology to remove unwanted hairs. Their marketing materials refer to this method of hair removal as achieving instant, painless results and long-lasting results.

Consumers beware. There have been no controlled studies on these devices. In my opinion, the results are no different than what you would achieve with shaving.

Pros: None.

Cons: You are paying a premium price for a device that functions similar to a shaver. The hairs are only removed at the surface level and will continue to grow. This is a short-term solution as the unwanted hairs will require continual maintenance.

Shaving
Manual | Disposable | Electric Razors

When using a manual or disposable razor, be sure to apply a lotion, foam or gel to the skin beforehand. Softening the hairs with a steam towel is also good idea; or you can just wait to shave at the end of a hot shower.

If your skin tends to become irritated from the act of shaving, apply a thin coating of Jojoba oil. This will work as a lubricant underneath the shaving cream as it will help the razor to glide more smoothly along the skin.

Pros: Shaving is easy, convenient and inexpensive. It can cover large areas quickly.

Cons: Shaving gives the hairs a blunt edge which feels somewhat prickly to the touch. Women have delicate facial skin which can become easily irritated and inflamed from shaving. It is also possible to develop breakouts and ingrown hairs after shaving the lip, chin and neck.

It is my opinion that <u>shaving should not be done on the face, neck, chest or stomach.</u> Even if you have terminal hairs in these areas, there is also a covering of fine vellus hairs. When these tiny hairs are tampered with, they will be stimulated to grow back longer, darker and more abundant over time.

Spring Coil Stick

This hand-held implement is rubbed along the surface of the skin in order to grab the hairs in its path.

Pros: It is inexpensive, reusable and capable of grabbing many hairs at a swipe. Also, it is very small and can be tucked away inside a makeup case in your handbag. You will get many sessions out of this implement before needing a replacement.

Cons: Although the action is similar to tweezing, it hurts more because so many hairs are being pulled out at the same time. Hairs must be at least 1/8" long in order to be grabbed by the spring coil stick.

Due to the pulling action of the coil, some of the thicker hairs may break off at the surface. It may also be necessary to go over the same area repeatedly in order to grab all the hairs.

This can cause redness, irritation and inflammation to the skin.

It is my opinion that the spring coil tool should not be used on the face, neck, chest or stomach. Even if you have terminal hairs in these areas, there is also a covering of fine vellus hairs. When these tiny hairs are tampered with, they will be stimulated to grow back longer, darker and more abundant over time.

Sugaring

Sugaring is a natural substance that is applied in a fashion similar to that of waxing. The sugaring compound can be mixed by hand using a combination of sugar, lemon juice and water until it reaches the correct consistency. Or it can be purchased readymade.

Sugaring is typically applied by hand and pressed firmly into the hairs. It is then pulled it off in the same direction that the hairs are growing.

Unlike waxing, there are no fabric strips or applicators needed.

Pros: This can be done at home or at a salon that features sugaring on their service menu. It is a natural product that is typically free of chemical components.

Sugaring is purported to be less painful than waxing. It is fine to use for hair removal on legs, arms, bikini and armpits.

Cons: Hair must be a minimum of 1/8" to 1/4" long in order to be removed with sugaring. This can cause some women embarrassment due to the visibility of the unwanted hairs.

It is my opinion that <u>sugaring should not be done on the face, neck, chest or stomach.</u> Even if you have terminal hairs in these areas, there is also a covering of fine vellus hairs. When these tiny hairs are tampered with, they will be stimulated to grow back longer, darker and more abundant over time.

Threading

Threading is an ancient form of hair removal that has been around for hundreds of years. It is practiced in India as well as many countries in the Middle East.

Threading is simplistic, yet fascinating to watch. A cotton thread is twisted in such a fashion so that it can grab the hairs out of the follicle as it rubs up against the skin.

Pros: It is quick, inexpensive and tidy. Threading is commonly performed on the eyebrows and facial areas, but can also be done on the body.

Cons: Each hair must have enough visible length (at least 1/8 of an inch) so that the thread can wrap around it, lasso-style, in order to yank it out. When the hairs are extremely thick, they may break off at the surface and then retract under the skin. The retracted hair can potentially become ingrown and trapped beneath the skin's surface.

When threading is done on a frequent basis (such as weekly or more) the skin may develop a red, rough surface in response to the continual irritation. For women with darker skin complexions, this also creates pigmentation which can look like a shadow or stain in areas such as the lip, chin and neck.

It is my opinion that <u>threading should not be done on the face, neck, chest or stomach.</u> Even if you have terminal hairs in these areas, there is also a covering of fine vellus hairs. When these tiny hairs are tampered with, they will be stimulated to grow back longer, darker and more abundant over time.

Tweezing

A tweezer is an implement used to pull out hairs individually. It is also handy in the removal of splinters.

Pros: Tweezing is an inexpensive method of removing bothersome hairs one by one. It is most often associated with eyebrow shaping.

Cons: In areas with a dense amount of hair growth, tweezing is a time-consuming undertaking.

Additionally, when the hairs are very thick and coarse, they sometimes break off at the surface while they are being pulled. The broken hair then retracts under the skin making it difficult to grab.

Some women are so determined to pull out the retracted hair that they end up digging into the skin causing bleeding, bruising and potential infection. When a scab forms over the hair, the hair will be trapped and often becomes ingrown.

Waxing

The goal of waxing is to pull the hair, in its entirety, out of the follicle. When the hair is pulled from the root, it can take several weeks for the root to regenerate and grow another hair to the skin's surface.

There are a variety of different wax types available on the market and they fall into three basic categories.

- Ready-to-use wax strips which may or may not need to be heated prior to use. They come already coated with the wax.
- Hot wax requires heat to soften it into a workable consistency. It is then spread evenly onto the skin with the use of an applicator such as a wooden stick. A piece of cloth is then firmly pressed into the wax and swiftly

ripped off the skin in an opposite direction from the hair growth.

- Hard wax is applied thickly and pulled off when it cools. No fabric strips are used with this method.

Pros: Waxing pulls the entire hair out of the skin from the root. It will take several days to a few weeks for all the hairs to be visible on the surface again. The reward is smooth skin that stays hair-free longer than shaving.

Cons: Depending upon the body part being waxed, positioning can be an issue when doing it yourself. For example, the back of the legs would be difficult to do by oneself. In this case, professional waxing at a salon would yield the best results.

Improper technique can cause bruising to the skin. Additionally, skin lifting and tearing can occur in individuals with thin fragile skin or those who use peeling agents.

Hair must be a minimum of 1/8" to 1/4" long in order to be waxed. This can cause some women embarrassment due to the visibility of the unwanted hairs.

It is my opinion that waxing should not be done on the face, neck, chest or stomach. Even if you have terminal hairs in these areas, there is also a covering of fine vellus hairs. When these tiny hairs are tampered with, they will be stimulated to grow back longer, darker and more abundant over time.

Note: With regard to the lower leg, I have noted a decrease in the amount of hair returning after many years of waxing. This is the only area of the body that seems to improve from repeated waxings.

All the hair on the lower leg is of the terminal variety. I believe that scar tissue may form over the root after years of repeated waxings.

I have also noted this phenomenon in the eyebrow region where the tweezed hairs are all terminal. I believe this explains why women who try to regrow and reshape their eyebrows often discover, to their dismay, that the original hairs rarely return.

Semi-Permanent Methods

Under ideal conditions -- fair skin and dark thick hairs -- a permanent reduction in the amount of hairs may be seen.

Permanent reduction means that many hair follicles will be disabled for life, while others will continue to produce replacement hairs with each new growth cycle.

Note: Melanin is a natural substance that is responsible for creating pigment in both the hair and the skin. It is produced by the melanocyte cells.

The shade of melanin in the hair as well as the skin will factor in to how effective the following semi-permanent methods will be.

IPL (Intense Pulsed Light)

This equipment uses an intensely concentrated light that targets melanin, the pigmentation which gives the hair its color.

The amount of melanin in our skin also determines how light or dark our skin tone will be.

IPL shines through the layers of the skin and converts to heat when it reaches its target, which in this case, is the melanin (pigmentation) in the hair.

In order to be most effective, the hair must be in the anagen stage of growth. During this phase, the hair remains attached to the bulb which is the root center of the follicle.

For best results, there must be a contrast between the hair color and the skin color. This means that candidates should have a light skin tone with dark hairs.

Pros: Fair-skinned women with dark hairs will see reduction in the amount of hair previously growing from the treated area. Hairs that regrow may return lighter in color and thinner in texture. Legs, bikini and underarms are the areas that achieve the best results.

Cons: Darker skin tones will not achieve optimal results. Plus the possibility of burning exists due to deeper pigmentation. Additionally, white and red hairs cannot be treated successfully.

Waxing and tweezing should not be done prior to the service. Sun exposure also must be avoided.

It is my opinion that <u>IPL should not be done on the face</u>.

When choosing this process, ask questions about training and experience of the technician. Also, inquire about third-party studies that have been conducted with regard to how IPL may affect the skin cells long-term.

Being an educated consumer will help you to make better choices.

Laser Hair Removal

LASER is an acronym which stands for "Light Amplification by Stimulated Emission of Radiation."

The laser shines a beam of highly concentrated light through the skin with the goal of targeting the hair root.

Keep the following three points in mind:

1. PIGMENT – The best chances for success with laser hair removal are achieved on light skin with dark thick hairs since the laser works by targeting pigment.
2. DENSITY – The greater the amount of dark hairs in a given area, the better the potential for reduced hair growth (i.e. armpit, bikini area, etc.)
3. SKIN THICKNESS – Thin skin tissue enables the laser light to penetrate deep enough into the skin to reach the

hair root and destroy it. Many women with light skin and dark thick hairs have good results on the bikini area since there is dense hair growth and the skin is thin.

Pros: If you have fair skin with dark dense hair growth, this would make you a good candidate for successful laser hair removal treatment. Best results are in the bikini area. Depending on the amount and distribution of hairs, there may be some improvement on arms, legs and armpits.

Cons: This procedure is expensive and multiple sessions are required. It is also somewhat painful.

It is my opinion that women should <u>never have laser hair removal done on the face</u>.

Note: Many women have noticed MORE hair growth on their faces after having had laser hair removal. This phenomenon is known as hypertrichosis and is caused by an increased blood supply to the hair root due to the heat of the laser.

Additionally, the face is typically shaved by the technician prior to the service. When tiny vellus hairs are tampered with, they are stimulated to grow back longer, darker and more abundant over time.

Laser seems to become less and less effective as the hairs thin out. Multiple treatments may possibly increase effectiveness, but the incremental improvement may not be worth the cost.

Darker complexions may experience pigmentation and burning from the laser.

There are many different types of lasers on the market. Results are dependent upon the body area being treated, the woman's skin and hair type as well as the skill of the technician.

When choosing this process, ask questions about the type of laser that will be used in your service as well as the training and experience of the technician. Also inquire about third-party studies that have been conducted with regard to how laser may affect the skin cells long-term.

Being an educated consumer will help you to make better choices.

Permanent Hair Removal

Permanent refers to the fact that once the hair root is completely destroyed, it will no longer be able to grow another hair.

Straight hair follicles are the easiest to treat and the fastest to achieve permanent removal.

Hairs that have been repeatedly tweezed, waxed, threaded and/or epilated, may cause the follicle to develop a curvature. In this case, the root may not be fully destroyed the first time and will need to be retreated with the next cycle of growth in order to achieve permanency.

Electrolysis

Electrolysis is performed using a thin wire called a probe that is gently inserted down the shaft of the hair follicle in order to concentrate heat on the hair root.

Keep the following three points in mind when comparing electrolysis to laser:

1. PIGMENT – Electrolysis can be done on any skin color, any skin type and any hair color.
2. DENSITY – Not a requirement for the success of electrolysis treatments.
3. SKIN THICKNESS – Thin or thick skin can be treated with equal results.

PROS: Electrolysis can be performed with great success on <u>all skin colors</u> {fair, tan, ethnic} and <u>all hair colors</u> {white, red, dark}.

Electrolysis can be done on any part of the body that has hair growth:

- Hairline
- Eyebrow
- Lip
- Chin
- Neck
- Cheeks
- Sideburns
- Chest
- Breast
- Stomach
- Bikini
- Legs
- Arms
- Fingers
- Toes

Electrolysis has been around for over a 100 years and has withstood the test of time for safety and permanence.

It is the ONLY method of hair removal that has been approved as "permanent" by the FDA.

Electrolysis can safely be used to shape eyebrows, redesign hairlines and permanently eradicate hairs remaining after countless laser sessions.

Cons: In order to achieve permanency, the client must stop other methods of hair removal such as tweezing, waxing and threading.

A firm commitment to the treatment schedule is necessary in order to achieve permanent results.

Electrolysis is more affordable than laser, but pricier than threading or waxing. However, after a set amount of treatments the hair will be removed permanently.

How does electrolysis work?

Each hair on the human body grows out of a follicle, which is a natural opening in the skin. The hair root is located at the bottom of this opening. Electrolysis functions to destroy the germinating root center so that a hair can no longer grow from the treated follicle.

A fine probe, thinner than the actual hair, is gently inserted down the shaft of the hair follicle. An experienced electrologist will note resistance as the probe encounters the root. At this precise juncture, an appropriate amount of heat will be emitted from the tip of the probe in order to destroy the growth center, rendering it unable to grow any future hairs. The hair is then lifted out of the treated follicle.

A large amount of individual hairs can be treated during an electrolysis session.

The length of the treatment is based upon the area requiring the work, the sensitivity of the skin and the tolerance of the client. Sessions can range from as little as 15 minutes to an hour or more.

Note: Electrolysis is a permanent process; however, it requires several sessions to treat all the hair growth cycles. Scheduling is determined based on the amount of hair present. Prior methods of hair removal influence how quickly results will be achieved.

Does it hurt?

Every woman experiences the sensation of electrolysis differently, and each area of the body has varying sensitivity. Most women comment that the treatments range from slightly bothersome to somewhat annoying.

Numbing creams are available for those that prefer them.

What if I have PCOS and high levels of androgens?

Once a hair root is fully destroyed by electrolysis, the treated follicle will no longer be capable of growing another hair. This means that the hair is permanently destroyed.

If a woman has extremely high levels of androgens, previously untreated follicles (typically consisting of fine vellus hairs) may begin to grow hairs that will become darker, thicker and longer in the future. This occurrence is due to androgens altering the hair root cells.

Androgen-sensitive hair growth is one of the many symptoms that women with PCOS deal with. In order to minimize future increases in new hair growth, it is important to consult with a physician in this regard. After testing, your doctor may determine that you require some form of hormonal therapy.

To reiterate, electrolysis will permanently eradicate hairs that grow from treated follicles, but it cannot prevent new hairs from growing out of untreated follicles in the future.

Women with androgen-sensitive hair growth will achieve more thorough clearance when electrolysis treatments are performed in conjunction with physician administered hormonal therapies.

How do I choose an electrolysis specialist?

When seeking the services of an electrologist, I encourage you to begin by scheduling an initial consultation. It is my firm belief that an understanding of the process is an important beginning to successful electrolysis treatment.

During the consultation, your new electrologist will evaluate your growth pattern in order to determine an appropriate and realistic treatment schedule. Prior methods of removal are taken into account as this information factors into how quickly your permanent hair removal results will be achieved.

Please note that your choice of an electrologist is absolutely paramount to the success of your treatments.

Search for a caring professional with years of experience who is sincerely passionate about helping you.

You will never regret having electrolysis, only that you didn't do it sooner!

Your Hair Removal Action Plan

Here are my suggestions for the most sensible ways to remove unwanted hairs per body area.

Note: For handy reference purposes, I have included a review of at the end of this section.

Choose one method from each category that is the best fit for you, your budget and your comfort level.

If you've read the prior chapters, you will understand why I do not endorse waxing, shaving or threading, etc. for the face.

Face (excluding eyebrow)
- Bleach
- Tweeze (only the worst hairs)
- Electrolysis

Eyebrows
- Tweeze
- Thread

- Waxing
- Electrolysis

Arms

- Bleach
- Waxing
- Sugaring
- Epilator
- Laser
- Electrolysis

Underarms

- Shaving
- Wax
- Sugaring
- Epilator
- Laser
- Electrolysis

Chest/Breasts

- Bleach
- Tweeze (only the worst hairs)
- Electrolysis

Stomach/Abdomen

- Bleach
- Electrolysis

Bikini

- Shaving
- Waxing
- Sugaring
- Laser
- Electrolysis

Legs

- Shaving
- Waxing
- Sugaring
- Epilator
- Laser
- Electrolysis

Fingers/Toes

- Bleach
- Shaving
- Waxing

- Sugaring
- Electrolysis

Hairline/Nape of Neck
- Electrolysis
- Tweezing

Review

Temporary Measures: Many may seem inexpensive, but actually cost more due to long-term use. Some are extremely inconvenient and bothersome.

>   Waxing, Threading, Tweezing, Shaving, Epilating, Depilatories, Bleaching and more

Semi-Permanent Measures: Some hair follicles will be disabled for life, while others will continue to produce replacement hairs with each new growth cycle.

>   IPL (Intense Pulsed Light) and Laser Hair Removal

Permanent: All treated hair follicles will stop producing hairs.

>   Electrolysis

Addendum

There are two additions that I've included below that were not covered earlier in the book:

Vaniqua® Prescription Cream

Vaniqua® is a cream available by prescription only. According to the manufacturer, this cream is capable of slowing the rate of hair growth. However, it does not permanently remove it. It is only designed for on the face.

Spearmint Tea

I am mentioning -- but NOT endorsing --this tea. It seems that some women with hormonal hair growth due to PCOS "claim" to have seen a reduction in hair growth after consuming it. I would advise you to confer with your physician before adding this to your diet. He or she will be able to check medical journals for studies in this regard.

Thank You

It has always been my passion to make a difference in people's lives.

I love my career and remain dedicated to helping women make better hair removal choices.

Thank you for you giving me this opportunity to educate and guide you.

Sincerely,

Lori Weintraub

Notes